MISOPHONIA
THE MENTAL DISORDER THAT MAKES ME HATE YOU

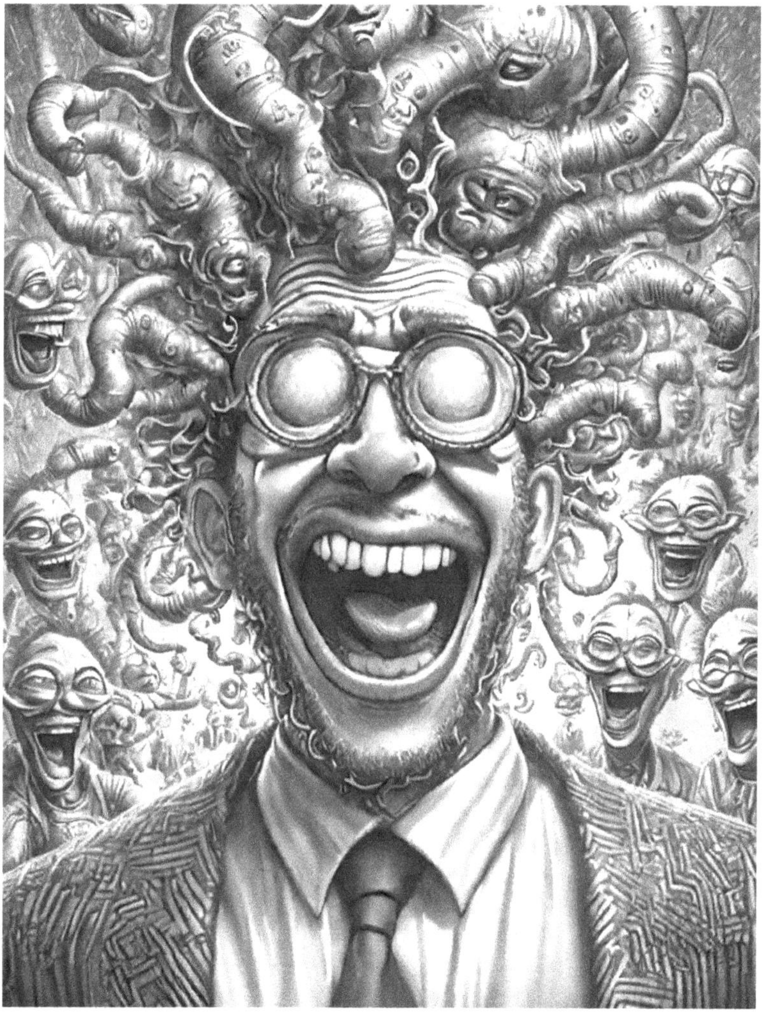

BRANDON BISHOP

MISOPHONIA

The Mental Disorder That Makes Me Hate You

BRANDON BISHOP

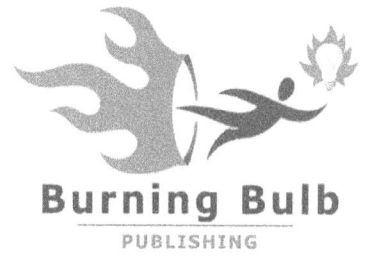

Misophonia: The Mental Disorder That Makes Me Hate You
By **Brandon Bishop**

Burning Bulb Publishing
P.O. Box 4721
Bridgeport, WV 26330-4721
United States of America
www.BurningBulbPublishing.com

Copyright © 2024 Brandon Bishop. All rights reserved.

Cover designed by Brandon Bishop.

First Edition.

Paperback Edition ISBN: 978-1-948278-91-1

Dedicated to every single one of you who "get" this book.

Yes, there are much worse illnesses and afflictions, but this is the one we share. There's no cure, no treatment, not even a real discussion for the most part… Just "Fight or Flight…"

Hopefully, you'll find some common ground in these pages and learn quickly that you're not the only one. Or maybe this will help you understand why you hate so many sounds and actions that others make. Or… Maybe you're living with someone who tells you to "Please chew with your mouth shut!" You might not even realize that you're basically torturing people around you.

Whatever the case, I hope this small token of understanding and promoted tolerance will offer some comfort or at least a nice distraction.

But yeah, "Please Chew with your mouth shut…"
We're begging you…

CHAPTER 1
WHAT IS MISOPHONIA?

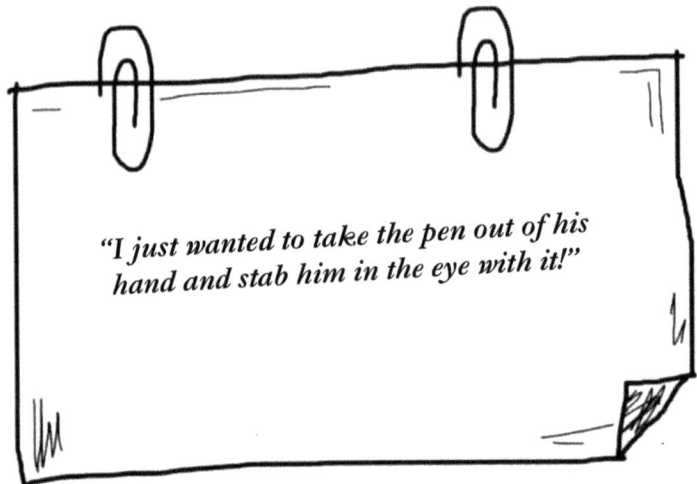

"I just wanted to take the pen out of his hand and stab him in the eye with it!"

That was a quote from one of the 6% of us that Misophonia really kicks the hell out of. While about 30% of Americans alone suffer from mild cases, the lucky number of 6% are driven to the brink of insanity on sometimes an hourly basis.

Misophonia. It's not merely a dislike for certain sounds; rather, it is an intense emotional reaction, an aversive response to specific auditory stimuli that can transform the everyday soundscape into an overwhelming cacophony. It's a rage-inducing hatred for any number of uncontrollable sounds caused, usually by other humans, sometimes by animals or nature, and even, in many cases, by one's self.

At its core, misophonia is characterized by heightened emotional reactions, ranging from discomfort to extreme distress, triggered by specific sounds. These annoying sounds, often referred to as "trigger noises," can vary widely among individuals but commonly include the likes of chewing, slurping, tapping, or even breathing sounds. While many of us may find such noises mildly irritating, those with misophonia experience an extreme and visceral response, leading to increased stress, anxiety, and often anger.

"You feel like you're trapped in hell," said one sufferer,

"I was stuck in a car with my grandparents, who I love so much, but once they started slurping on these caramel candies and smacking their lips, I just wanted to get out of the car and run away…"

That quote reminds me of my own earliest days of dealing with this crap. I doubt the term Misophonia existed in any medical journals at that time in the 80s.

My stepdad, at the time, was a good man. I haven't spoken with him in decades at this point, and that's fine, but he took my mom and me out of the slums of Detroit and into the suburbs. I'll always be grateful to Frank for that, and I wish we still had some form of contact so I could at least thank him for what he did for our family back then.

But… He drove me crazy. Not for any fault of his own; he was clueless. But that line above about the chewy caramels… He loves those things. I recall one long drive in his truck; I immediately saw the bag of chewy candy right by his side and pondered my punishment for grabbing them and tossing them out the window. I'm sure it would've been worth it.

It was a long drive out to some hunting field he was checking out, and I was in tow for some reason. I think we were forcing ourselves to get along, you know, "stepdad" stuff. I've been there; it's always awkward. But I forgot to bring my Walkman and headphones and a nice supply of hair metal tapes to fill my ears with anything but the horrid sound of this man chewing those caramels one after another. I buried my head in my jacket with my ears growing sore from inserted fingers. Just the peripheral image of his bearded jaw moving up and down and mouth hanging open drove me insane. On top of that, he whistled when he breathed through his nose. It was pure hell, and I didn't know why.

Again, this is not HIS fault whatsoever. He's chewing a piece of candy and breathing, for freak's sake. I knew if I asked him, even respectfully and kindly, "Could you not smack your lips while chewing those things…" I just knew it wouldn't end so well. I'm not saying he'd beat my ass or anything; he never did that, but either I'd piss him off, or he take offense or something.

So, for several hours, I was in a completely silent rage. I started eating the caramel myself to empty the bag faster. I must've eaten 10 of those sugar bombs.

It's funny how our brains work, isn't it? That could've been and MIGHT have been a fun little day in a Michigan forest, step dad and step son getting to know each other and spending some quality time on a road trip together... but no... I hated every mile and every minute of that trip. While in the quiet woods, I kept my distance from his heavy breathing.

Looking back now, it makes me angry. I haven't had a father figure like him before or since. He was in my life for over 20 years, and instead of being able to embrace him fully, instead of having a DAD in my life that I looked up to and wanted to spend time with, I had a guy that I'd avoid at every meal or snack, or basically, anytime he was breathing. Misophonia took that from me.

My mom is my best friend...Now... Back then, she was the other side of the torture duo I lived with. There were also two things my mom did that drove a wedge between us and put me on the outs with her as well.

She wasn't nearly as barbaric as an eater as Frank was, but she did more than her share of lip-smacking. Thanksgiving often saw me sit between them both during our old-school family dinners. It was like a stereo symphony of the loudest chewing I had heard. It was brutal. As much as I LOVE some juicy turkeys and all the fixings, I'd power eat through the meal (Quietly, of course) and leave the table. Thanksgiving was the worst. Often, I'd sneak into the kitchen where all the food was and pick and munch in there, far away from the Vikings and Mongols at the crowded table. I had to! Again, it's not their fault!

My mom would also, at that time, thankfully not these days, pronounce her letter "S's" with the highest screaming brat stabbing pitch possible. I swear dogs in other neighborhoods would be tilting their heads in curiosity when my mom was hitting those "S's" hard on the phone.

I'd be up in my room with the TV on, the fan going, the radio on, and my head buried in a blanket, and I'd still hear very "Ss... Sssssss... Ssssss...." In her conversation.

Again, she doesn't do any of this stuff now. Outside of the occasional somewhat tolerable dry mouth lip smack, I enjoy hanging out with the mom as much as possible. Like I said, she's my very best friend, and I love our time together. When the lip smacks get too frequent, I just leave. Fight or flight, and I'll never fight my mom. (I'd lose...)

I think back to those days, and I have a ton of regrets. I had good parents. I had a good life. I should have embraced them and treated them like royalty for what they did for me. And it's easy to SAY that at age 50 right now, regrets are always simple to erase in hindsight verbally. But I couldn't stand it. It hurt... and it's a pain that never went away, not even to this day... and if anything, it's gotten so much worse...

CHAPTER 2
THE CATALYSTS OF DISCOMFORT: CAUSES OF MISOPHONIA

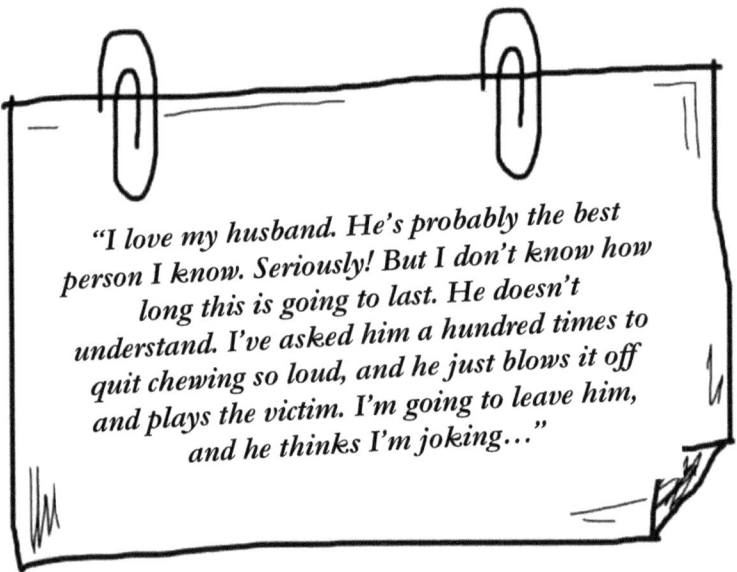

"I love my husband. He's probably the best person I know. Seriously! But I don't know how long this is going to last. He doesn't understand. I've asked him a hundred times to quit chewing so loud, and he just blows it off and plays the victim. I'm going to leave him, and he thinks I'm joking..."

Figuring out the mystery of misophonia involves exploring its origins. Researchers and clinicians have identified many potential factors contributing to the "Fight or Flight" intense reaction. Here's the scientific research stuff you've all been waiting for. Let me do my best to sound professional and pretend like I know what I'm talking about.

1. **Auditory Processing Differences:**
Individuals with misophonia may exhibit differences in how their brains process auditory stimuli. Certain sounds, often repetitive or patterned, may be processed differently, triggering strong emotional responses.

2. Emotional Conditioning:

The association between specific sounds and negative emotions plays a crucial role in misophonia. Early negative experiences linked to particular noises can create a conditioned response, where the brain perceives these sounds as threats, leading to heightened emotional reactions.

3. Neurobiological Factors:

Neurological studies suggest that misophonia might be linked to the central nervous system's hyper-activation. The limbic system, responsible for emotions, and the autonomic nervous system may be hypersensitive in individuals with misophonia, contributing to the severity of their reactions.

4. Genetic Predisposition:

There is evidence to suggest a genetic component to misophonia. Individuals with a family history of misophonia may be more prone to developing the condition, pointing to a genetic predisposition that influences one's sensitivity to certain sounds.

5. Cognitive Factors:

Cognitive processes, such as attention and selective focus, play a role in the perception of trigger sounds. Individuals with misophonia often exhibit an increased awareness of and attention to specific noises, intensifying their emotional response.

6. Control:

In my opinion, a lack of control element plays a factor in our discomfort and dislike of these noises. We can't always make them stop, whether it is a drip from the faucet, someone humming, or turning pages in a book. We immediately weigh our options for intervening against weighing our own discomfort for leaving the situation.

Understanding misophonia requires a holistic approach, considering the interplay of psychological, neurological, and environmental factors. It is not a mere aversion to irritating sounds but a complex interweaving of biology, psychology, and personal history. As science digs deeper into the realm of this audio-sensory issue, we begin to appreciate the intricacies of this unique symphony of discomfort and the challenges faced by those of us who navigate it in our daily lives.

Thankfully, in recent years, Misophonia has hit the trendy topic ledger for colleges and scientific studies across the board.

Prominent institutions and experts have spearheaded investigations into the neurological, psychological, and genetic aspects of misophonia.

Department of Psychology, Newcastle University:

Notably, the work led by researchers at Newcastle University's Department of Psychology has shed light on the neurobiological underpinnings of misophonia. Studies have explored brain imaging techniques to understand how the brain processes trigger sounds and why certain noises evoke such intense emotional responses.

Duke University:

Researchers at Duke University have delved into the genetic components of misophonia. Their work has suggested that misophonic reactions may have a hereditary aspect, with specific individuals being more genetically predisposed to developing heightened sensitivity to specific sounds.

Emory University:

At Emory University, investigations into the limbic system's role in misophonia have provided valuable insights. Understanding the emotional processing mechanisms in individuals with misophonia has been a focal point, with implications for potential therapeutic interventions.

And several other reputable institutions have been sinking their wisdom teeth into Misophonia. I'm not sure they're confident about finding a cure or a treatment, but they're curious... Curious is good, right?

CHAPTER 3
THE SOUNDS OF HATE

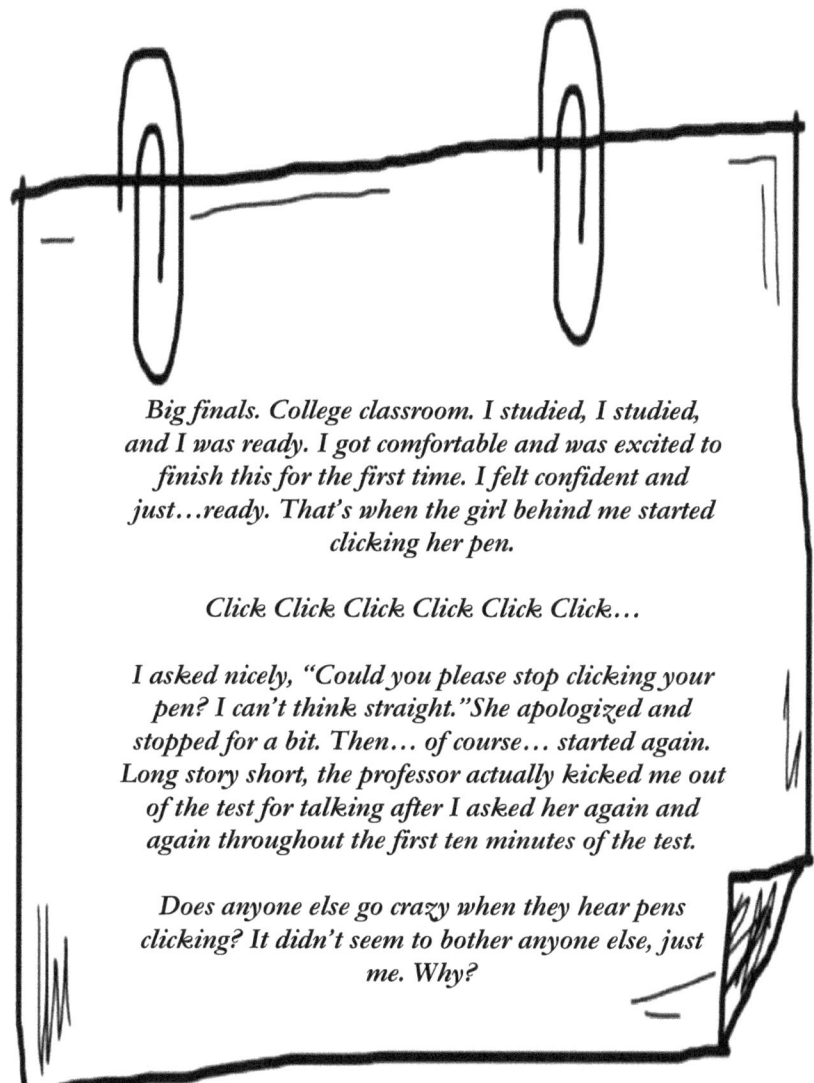

Big finals. College classroom. I studied, I studied, and I was ready. I got comfortable and was excited to finish this for the first time. I felt confident and just…ready. That's when the girl behind me started clicking her pen.

Click Click Click Click Click Click…

I asked nicely, "Could you please stop clicking your pen? I can't think straight." She apologized and stopped for a bit. Then… of course… started again. Long story short, the professor actually kicked me out of the test for talking after I asked her again and again throughout the first ten minutes of the test.

Does anyone else go crazy when they hear pens clicking? It didn't seem to bother anyone else, just me. Why?

Well, the answer is a resounding "YES!" I also had that same situation in college with a pen clicker, and I was asked to keep my voice down, but ultimately, I got up and left. Thankfully, it wasn't a test day, though.

I HATED school! Funny enough, Grade school and even High School were okay. I don't remember anyone annoying me to death in those grades. But once I was all grown up and in college, yeah. EVERYBODY drove me nuts! I had to sit in the very back row to avoid having anyone in the seats behind me. Suppose I heard breathing or pens clicking or chewing or lisping or crinkling papers; that was it. I was leaving.

The list of various sounds that drive us crazy is diverse and perpetually endless. What bothers me might not bother you. While everyone should hate and verbally SHAME those who chew loudly and smack their lips, it does not bother others with misophonia; in some countries like South Korea, I think it's customary and widely encouraged to lip smack while chewing. I spent a year in the Army, and I'll tell you this... I had many Korean friends and shared many meals with many of them. They're the worst. It's just straight-up smacking, every bite, every chew, every couple of seconds. Pure hell. I love Korea; I can't wait to go back, but holy shit, I hope their customs have been altered to rid the atmosphere of that rhythmic smacking.

If I had a group of Korean friends with me while having a meal, it would sound like ten horses trotting through a massive pool of Mac & cheese. I'm serious! It's just the worst!

So, what are some other classic Misophonia-related sounds that drive us absolutely batty? Well, I have a list. I'll toss out some popular Misophonia hatreds with a brief description and then give you my personal take. Here we go...

1. Chewing Gum Popping:
The rhythmic popping of chewing gum triggers an immediate fight-or-flight response, causing distress for individuals with misophonia.

It's the OG of all horrible sounds. We will never understand why people insist on doing this. It just doesn't make a SLURP of sense. It's gross and, in our opinion, disrespectful. CHEW WITH YOUR MOUTH SHUT! I host a TV show called "Go There Eat That" on ASY TV and have filmed at over 100 restaurant locations nationwide.

NOT ONCE can you find a single solitary lip smack. If I can do it, so can you!

2. Pen Clicking:

The constant clicking of a pen, whether in a meeting or a quiet library, becomes an unbearable stimulus for those with misophonia. The sharp, repetitive sound elicits heightened anxiety and frustration, making concentration nearly impossible.

Like I just said, it ruins concentration, and we start to fantasize about stabbing people with said pens. It's not okay.

3. Sniffling:

The continuous sniffling of an individual with a cold can be torture for those with misophonia. The repetitive nature of the sound exacerbates irritation, leading to an overwhelming urge to escape the environment.

Even when I'm doing it myself on the rare occasion, I find myself ill. It drives us crazy, doesn't it? You want to yell out, "Blow your Effin' Nose!"

4. Throat Clearing:

The repetitive act of throat clearing is a trigger that can induce extreme annoyance for individuals with misophonia. Whether in a workplace or social setting, the noise heightens stress levels and prompts a strong negative response.

Now, I know it's something that starts happening when you get older; hell, I do it now. This one doesn't bug me too badly, but after a while, depending on the quiet levels of the room and the volume of throat clearing... Yeah... Ugh...

5. Loud Breathing:

Audible or heavy breathing becomes a source of intense agitation for those with misophonia. The proximity of the sound can lead to heightened anxiety, pushing individuals to seek escape and refuge from the distressing noise.

I was whistling while breathing kills me, as I mentioned with my former stepdad. But also heavy breathing. I do a YouTube vlog called The ASY TV LIFE, and sometimes, when I'm watching old episodes back where I'm walking, all I can hear is my own breathing, which drives me stupid.

6. Nail Tapping:

The rhythmic tapping of nails on surfaces intensifies stress for those with misophonia. Whether it's on a desk or another hard surface, the sound triggers an immediate reaction.

I was on a trip from Colorado Springs to New Orleans. The lady sitting next to me while I was driving was and IS a great friend, BUT... She was non-stop texting for the entire road trip with her long acrylic nails. Every letter pressed on her phone was a "click." Even though it was her Minivan we were driving, I wanted to push her out of it while on the highway. People, THINK! I ask myself constantly, "Am I annoying anyone?" It's called being respectful. If you do ask yourself that question in public or around others, you're an asshole.

7. Silverware Scraping Plates:

The scraping of silverware against plates during a meal is a prominent misophonia trigger. The high-pitched, grating noise can induce an overwhelming emotional response, prompting affected individuals to seek a quieter space.

I don't hear this much. But I can only imagine when I do, it'll hit me right in the spine. It's the old-school chalkboard screech. It's terrible, but thankfully, it's rarely repetitive.

8. Foot Tapping:

The repetitive tapping of feet, especially in quiet environments, can drive individuals with misophonia to the edge. The persistent nature of the sound heightens irritation, causing an urgent need to distance oneself from the source.

Oh man, I'm guilty of this on every level. As a drummer for my entire life, I beat everything. I try to limit it around others, but I catch myself doing it constantly. So, I humbly apologize to anyone I've annoyed with my masterful beats. It does burn calories, though. And it keeps in time as a human. So, I have my reasons. But yeah, sorry about that.

9. Keyboard Typing:

The repetitive and rhythmic noise of keyboard typing, particularly in a quiet workspace, can induce stress for individuals with misophonia. The constant sound becomes a source of distraction, hindering concentration.

It's funny; as I'm typing this on the old MacBook Pro, I'm wondering if anyone downstairs can hear this. I'm currently staying with my Mom and her husband as he's going through cancer treatments and all that comes with it. I would hate to noise pollute the house with my rapid typing. They haven't said anything yet, so hopefully, I'm being a stealthy writer.

10. Page Turning:

The sound of pages turning, especially in a library or other quiet setting, can be distressing for those with misophonia. The delicate nature of the sound exacerbates irritation, making it difficult to focus on other tasks.

This one doesn't bother me whatsoever. I consider that sounds relaxing to be honest. But... I can see how others would hate this. I imagine a kid with the Miso sitting at the dinner table with his mom or dad, rifling through the newspaper and loudly fanning each page as he adjusts it and moves into another section. But thankfully, it is not a hindrance in my world.

11. Snoring:

The persistent sound of snoring, especially in close quarters, can be a significant trigger for individuals with misophonia. The rhythmic nature of the noise can disrupt sleep and intensify feelings of frustration.

This has ended relationships. I used to snore terribly, but for whatever reason, I just stopped. I only snore now if I'm in a strange bed or too hot, but overall, I'm grateful not to wake up with a sore throat these days.

But when it comes to sleeping or being around others that snore loudly. Yeah, it isn't very pleasant. I'm unsure if this falls under Misophonia guidelines, but it can undoubtedly be rage-inducing.

I've been guilty of the subtle "Nudge" to snorers, all the way up to making loud noise to wake them or even impromptu pillow fights.

12. Finger Snapping:
The sudden and sharp sound of finger snapping can induce an immediate stress response in individuals with misophonia. The unpredictability of the noise heightens discomfort, leading to a strong adverse reaction.

I don't know about this one, either. I mean, if someone is standing near me, snapping their fingers for 5 minutes. I'll ask them nicely, "What the hell are you doing???" But how many times does this really happen?

13. Velcro Ripping:
The distinct sound of Velcro ripping apart becomes a significant trigger for those with misophonia. The sharp, tearing noise intensifies irritation, prompting an urgent desire to avoid the source.

Again, it doesn't phase me unless someone is just doing it over and over again for no good reason. If I worked at a jacket factory and the person beside me was doing their job by ripping apart velcro, I can't see that driving me up the wall. Plus, headphones…Headphones are a saving grace.

14. High Heel Clicking:
The rhythmic clicking of high heels on hard surfaces can be distressing for individuals with misophonia. The repetitive nature of the sound exacerbates discomfort, making it challenging to tolerate.

Yeah… this one. I understand the need and want to look sexy. And yes, high heels are fashionable and work for some. Yet… In a long tile, floored echoes office building on an 8-hour shift, and they're walking past your desk every 5 minutes. I'd contemplate tripping…

15. Trucks, Microwaves and other Beeping:
Repetitive beeping, especially in a quiet place, can be a significant trigger for individuals with misophonia. The constant noise becomes irritating, prompting a strong negative reaction.

Microwaves don't bother me. They give off maybe 4-5 reps, and then it's over. That goes for most beeping situations. But construction sites…

The constant sounds of trucks and bulldozers backing up again and again and again are mind-numbing. It's even worse when they're working on your street, and you can hear it over and over in your own house. Thankfully, it only lasts a few days to a couple weeks normally, and for as long as they work on those particular days. But those are NOT good days.

Allow me to throw in roofers here as well. The constant, seemingly never-ending nail guns are enough to drive me and most pets insane.

16. Shoe Squeaking:

The squeaking of shoes, particularly on polished floors, becomes a distressing noise for those with misophonia.

This is another one I cannot stand hearing while I'm doing it. Other people usually walk by quickly, and it's not a big deal at all. But when I'm stuck listening to my own squeaky shows, it makes me just want to go barefoot.

17. Water Dripping:

The persistent sound of water dripping, especially in a quiet space, becomes a source of heightened anxiety for those with misophonia. The rhythmic nature of the noise can be overwhelming, prompting a strong emotional response.

Thankfully there are methods to ending a leaking faucet. But when a drip is coming from outside your window at night, or maybe from an unknown location. It can trigger massive anger.

18. Birds

While generally pleasant, the constant chirping of birds, especially when disruptive, can trigger heightened anxiety for individuals with misophonia. The proximity of the noise amplifies irritation, prompting an immediate stress response.

I love the sounds of chirping birds. Until I don't...

19. Barking Dogs:

The persistent barking of dogs, particularly in a quiet neighborhood, can be a significant trigger for those with misophonia. The repetitive nature of the sound intensifies discomfort, making it challenging to find relief.

I can't count the number of times I've said to myself, "Who's barking dog is that? Why are they just ignoring it?" I've never had a dog. I like dogs, but Misophonia won't allow me to listen to them drinking water or licking themselves constantly. It was bad enough with Marci J Cat.

I had Marci for almost 19 years before she passed on February 11th, 2023, from cancer. I loved that mower with all of my heart, but when she drank water or cleaned herself, I had to distance myself. Dogs are 100 times louder in those aspects. And they BARK! If my dog were outside barking for 10 minutes straight, I'd get out there and scope the scene and then tell it to quit. It's simple, right? Some of you shitty dog owners just let them go for hours... I don't get it.

20. Cell Phones:

The sudden and loud ringing of phones, especially in quiet environments, can induce stress for individuals with misophonia. The abruptness of the sound disrupts concentration, prompting a strong negative reaction.

Okay... I've tried to keep the swearing to a minimum. I honestly never use profane language in public or in my books, but on this topic, I may allow a few to slip through my personal filters.

First, Unless you're deaf or expecting an important or emergency call or text, If you live with others... TURN YOUR RINGER OFF! No one else enjoys hearing that you're getting texts, calls, and notifications all day. It's extremely rude and disrespectful to subject anyone to your cell phone sounding off all day and night. TURN IT OFF!

Secondly, " If you're in public or around other people in general, and you feel the need to entertain yourself by watching Instagram videos or Facebook Reels or TikTok's or whatever they call that crap, WEAR HEADPHONES or KEEP THE VOLUME OFF or TO A MINIMUM!

This is a huge pet peeve of mine. And that's basically what Misophonia gives us: a list of what we used to call simple "Pet Peeves."

Nothing puts me in a fight or flight status more than when people at the airport, at a restaurant, or in a house just BLARE what they're watching on their phone. It's horribly disrespectful, and everyone around you HATES it. STOP FREAKIN' DOING THAT!

I was at a doctor's appointment a few weeks before I wrote this. Just a simple yearly check-up to ensure everything is still moving and grooving. In the waiting room, there was this dipshit BLASTING some ghetto ass video with people arguing and fighting, followed by my terrible mumble rap "music," followed by more drama and negativity and bad music. AT A DOCTOR'S OFFICE WAITING ROOM with five other people sitting there glaring at him. WHAT AN ASSHOLE!

Since we're not legally allowed to punch people in the throat anymore, all I could do is leave. I guarantee that if I respectfully and politely asked him to turn his volume off, he'd enter victim mode and start a scene. I don't have time or patience for that, nor did I feel like sitting in a jail cell over some worthless disrespectful shithead. So I walked away.

Sometimes that's the best option, isn't it? Just leave. Pick FLIGHT over FIGHT, no matter how desperately you want to twist them into a salty pretzel. It's not worth it.

Managing my anger caused by Misophonia and all-around stupid people has been a long work process. I'm getting better, but man... not too much better.

21. Crunching Ice:

The sharp and repetitive sound of ice crunching, especially in close quarters, becomes distressing for those with misophonia. The proximity of the sound intensifies irritation, prompting an immediate stress response.

Go hand in hand with loud eating. Yet, I don't hear this much, and it doesn't bug me when I do it. But I can quickly see how others would hate it, especially if they're around someone who constantly chews ice.

22. Ticking Clocks:

The rhythmic ticking of clocks, particularly in a quiet room, can be distressing for individuals with misophonia. The constant noise becomes a source of irritation, making it challenging to focus on other tasks.

This one... yeah... I love Grandfather Clocks and Glockenspiels. I think antique clocks are beautiful, and I would love to have many around the house... But no...

I was at an Antique market in Colorado and saw one of the coolest Grandfather-style clocks I've ever seen. It was solid black, looked like a coffin, and had silver chains for bells; it was just the coolest thing ever. I saw that it was only 199 bucks, and right then and there, I said to myself, "This is mine forever..."

I asked someone to help me with it and waited for them to grab a cart to take it out to my van. While waiting, it got quiet. I noticed the rhythmic ticking emanating from this amazing piece of art. Then, behind it were several other clocks, all ticking per second. I honestly had a mini meltdown that lasted about 4 seconds, but that was plenty.

The guy showed up with the clock, and I had to inform him that I had changed my mind. I opted for a smaller awl clock in the same design. This one also ticked, but I removed the battery and hung it as a work of art.

23. Loud Sneezing:

The sudden and loud sneezing of an individual, wildly when unexpected, can trigger heightened anxiety for those with misophonia. The abruptness of the sound disrupts the surrounding environment, intensifying the emotional response.

I mean, people sneeze. It's quick and usually painless. I always sneeze twice; some people sneeze forty times, and it's crazy loud. While it can be somewhat unpleasant, especially if they don't cover their mouths and nose, this one doesn't kill me in any way. You?

24. Coughing:

Prolonged and loud coughing fits, especially in confined spaces, become a significant source of distress for those with misophonia. The continuous nature of the noise intensifies irritation, making it challenging to tolerate.

I hate it. I lived with my Grandma for about two years; she smoked like a chimney. It eventually killed her and others I love. I hate smoking. But, of course, coughing doesn't come solely from smoking.

Either way, constant coughing, and hacking are just the worst. When I'm doing it, it's terrible because I hate coughing like anyone does and because I don't want to annoy others around me.

When smokers or potheads are hacking, I wouldn't say I like it because smoking is stupid, and not only do I have to smell that garbage, but now I get to enjoy a symphony of coughs.

When someone is sick and coughing, I tend not to hate it as much, but LOUD and UNCOVERED coughs are just cringy.

25. Whistling:

The sudden and sharp sound of whistling, especially in a quiet setting, can induce an immediate stress response for individuals with misophonia. The unpredictability of the noise heightens discomfort, prompting a strong negative reaction.

There was this lady a few years back at a Salvation Army Thrift Store whistling Christmas music so loudly that the entire packed store turned on her. This lady thought she was on stage at Carnegie Hall entertaining the masses with her unbelievably loud whistling.

Of course, she was clueless about why about four people gave her the cold shoulder treatment and exhaled loudly in annoyance around her. She blurted out, "What?" To a lady shaking her head slowly at her. I chimed in, of course, "The whistling… It's loud and terrible, and you've been doing it for the entire time I've been in this place." "I'm just trying to spread some Christmas spirit!" I think she responded in so many words. "Well, you failed and ruined the holidays for everyone here…" I joked. Thankfully, she and everyone else laughed, and all was right in the world. We were even more thankful that she quit whistling.

26. Motorcycles:

The loud and sudden revving of a motorcycle engine, especially in close proximity, can trigger heightened anxiety for individuals with misophonia. The abruptness of the sound disrupts the surrounding environment, intensifying the emotional response.

Sorry, biker dudes, you're not that cool anymore. After South Park roasted bikers, I hoped they'd trade in their leather vests and choppers and quit annoying everyone… but sadly, no… they still dress up in biker costumes and rev their engines in the most inopportune locations.

Thankfully, ill call it the "Biker Fart" sound comes and goes quickly as a great deal of them ride like complete assholes. But we all HATE that neighbor down the street with the loud-ass motorcycle. He cares very little that everyone in town can hear him start it up and rev down the street. It's insufferable.

27. Fireworks Explosions:

The loud explosions of fireworks, wildly when unexpected, can induce an immediate stress response for individuals with misophonia.

Let's chat my overtly and moronic patriotic friends.

It's called The FOURTH of July. On this day, it's highly acceptable to pop off a few cool fireworks, sparklers, etc. Have a fun family BBQ, down those processed meats, and drown yourself in alcohol, all in the name of whatever freedom you truly believe you have. Do it... Have fun! But maybe keep it between 7 pm and 10 pm. Is that fair? I think most elderly people, babies, pets, and those with PTSD would agree. But these people don't care about that! MEAT! BEER! FIREWORKS! MEAT! BEER! FIREWORKS! MEAT! BEER! FIREWORKS! They are just horrible and disrespectful wastes of flesh.

But let's get back to my original point. It's the FOURTH of July... No one celebrates The 2nd, 3rd, 5th, 6th, or any other day in July. Pop off your crap on the 4th and wrap it up til next year. OR... Just go to a fireworks show in town. I used to love those! Yours are not going to be better.

28. Movie Theaters:

It's the worst. Picture the scene. You're in a movie theater. The movie starts... You've been waiting long and paid a pretty hefty ticket price to watch this film. And then it starts... The crinkling of plastic candy wrappers, the open mouth chewing of buttery popcorn, the slurping of sugary drinks and the sounds the straw makes moving in and out of the plastic lid, the constant chatter of thoughtless people trying to figure out the plot, phones going off, kids crying, etc., etc., etc.

I used to love going to the movies. A theater visit was something I looked forward to all week. And yes, today, theaters are getting better. In the nicer ones, you're not sitting an ice away from someone. Some theaters have recliners and trays, and every seat in the house is a good one. I can stomach those... But the other old-school ghetto theaters are a thing of my past. Misophonia will not allow it.

29. Wanna Be Lawn Professionals:

The loud and continuous noise of a lawn mower or leaf blower, especially in close proximity, can induce stress for individuals with misophonia. The constant nature of the noise becomes a source of irritation, prompting an immediate stress response.

I'm not talking about the actual lawn care services that come and go within 30 minutes and do a great job. I'm talking about the DUDES (it's always men.) who have found a viable escape from their miserable lives inside the house by mowing their tiny lawns for hours 4 times a week. They only have a small strip of grass, and they're out there for hours! I don't get it.

Then, fall comes, and the leaves descend from the trees. Here, they come in full overcompensation mode... The Leaf Blowers.

Guys, You're basically holding a gas-powered engine that everyone can hear for blocks in every direction. Sure, blow your leaves into a pile and get it done. There is NO REASON to be out there daily blowing leaves around. Better yet... Grab a RAKE! Remember those? They burn calories, and you can stay away from your family even longer.

I'm just trying to help...

30. Babies:

The sound of a baby crying, especially when persistent, can trigger heightened anxiety for those with misophonia. The constant nature of the noise becomes a source of irritation, making it challenging to tolerate.

My days of raising babies or screaming, annoying kids in general are over. NEVER AGAIN!

Thankfully, my son Brandon Jr. never really cried, never really threw a fit, or acted like a complete mess of a tiny human. I was lucky. I saw and dated others with the shittiest kids imaginable, which has a great deal to do with why I'm single today and probably always will be.

When a baby starts crying, it triggers the knowledge that I'm stuck with it. And I hate that feeling. You can't punch a baby; you just can't... You can't even really tell it to shut its face. It's even more taboo to ask the parents to keep it quiet. Most parents are dealing with it at ground zero as well.

But yeah, a baby can hit all the painful points in your brain with a good howling. No more babies, nope!

31. Car Sounds:

The constant idling of a car engine, especially when in close proximity, becomes a significant trigger for individuals with misophonia. The persistent noise becomes a source of irritation, prompting an immediate stress response.

I live a great deal of my life in my van. I sleep by highways, in parking lots, gas stations, Cracker Barrel, you name it. The sound of traffic never really bothers me. But car alarms, Loud idling trucks, gas-powered generators from RVs, losers blasting BASS music from their systems, constant revving engines, motorcycles (again), douchebags squealing tires while drag racing at stoplights, people talking loudly on Bluetooth car devices, and so many other things… yeah… it can push a man with the vicious MISO into insanity.

Listen, I could go on and on with the list of 200 sounds and situations I researched that place Misophoniacs into a rage of sorts, but I think I covered most of the greatest hits. Some other some, others bother others. Such is the case in all of humanity; no two of us are the same.

If I left anything off that truly pokes at your tolerance and abilities to withstand, look up the Facebook Page, and we can discuss it there. I'm sure there's a long, long list out there that I never even thought of.

CHAPTER 4
BUT IS IT CLINICAL YET?

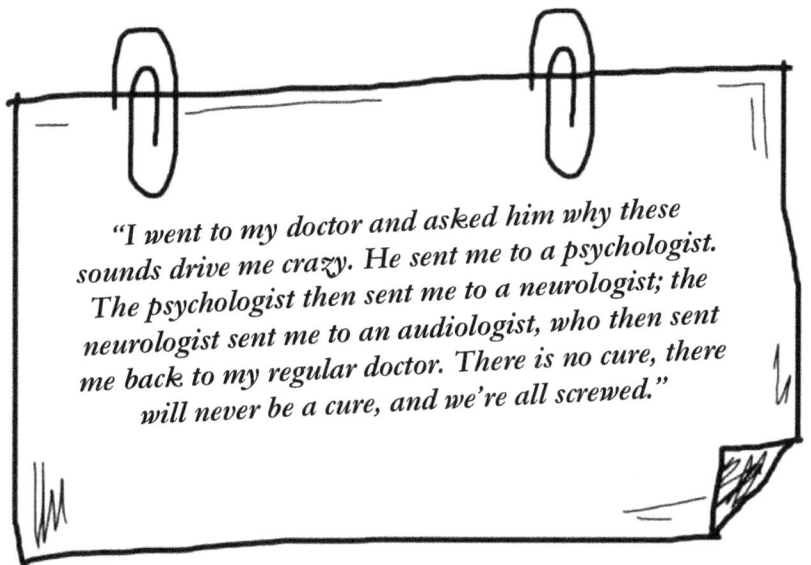

"I went to my doctor and asked him why these sounds drive me crazy. He sent me to a psychologist. The psychologist then sent me to a neurologist; the neurologist sent me to an audiologist, who then sent me back to my regular doctor. There is no cure, there will never be a cure, and we're all screwed."

I can so relate. I often imagine living a life where this stuff doesn't phase me at all. Where I could have eaten with my parents as a kid, where the lady behind me on the airplane with the blistering "SSSSSS's" doesn't literately hurt the center of my brain. But has any work gone into studying this?

Let's talk all clinical and professionally again.

The clinical diagnosis of misophonia is a nuanced process that involves collaboration between clinicians, audiologists, and mental health professionals. Individuals seeking assistance often undergo comprehensive assessments to evaluate their auditory sensitivities, emotional responses, and overall impact on daily functioning.

1. Diagnostic Criteria:
While misophonia is not yet officially recognized as a distinct psychiatric disorder in widely accepted diagnostic manuals such as the

DSM-5, its impact on mental health and daily life is increasingly acknowledged. Clinicians rely on self-reporting trigger sounds, emotional responses, and functional impairments to guide their evaluations.

2. Questionnaires and Interviews:
Clinicians may employ specialized questionnaires and structured interviews to gather detailed information about an individual's experiences with misophonia. These tools help assess the severity of symptoms, the range of trigger sounds, and the emotional toll on the individual's well-being.

3. Collaborative Approaches:
A multidisciplinary approach involving psychologists, audiologists, and neuroscientists is often employed to understand misophonia holistically. This collaborative effort enhances diagnostic accuracy and facilitates a more comprehensive understanding of the condition.

***

So, will there ever be a cure? Is being annoyed by other people and sometimes by myself even a curable issue?

The quest for a cure for misophonia remains an ongoing challenge. While scientific advancements have illuminated various aspects of the condition, developing a universally effective cure is complicated by the varied nature of misophonic experiences. Again, what bugs me may not bug you, etc.

1. Therapeutic Interventions:
Current approaches to managing misophonia focus on coping strategies and therapeutic interventions. Cognitive-behavioral therapy (CBT), sound therapy, and exposure therapy are methods employed to help individuals mitigate their emotional responses and improve daily functioning. I don't think this will help. I'm willing to try anything, but trying to make me get USED TO these sounds might kill me in the process.

2. Neuroscientific Advances:

As neuroscientific understanding progresses, there is hope that targeted interventions based on neural mechanisms may emerge. Yet, the complexity of the brain's response to trigger sounds poses challenges in developing a one-size-fits-all solution.

3. Genetic and Pharmacological Exploration:

I don't know how any of this could be genetic, but research into the genetic basis of misophonia may open avenues for personalized treatments in the future. Pharmacological interventions that modulate neurobiological processes associated with misophonia are also areas of interest, though substantial research is needed to establish their findings. Of course, BIG PHARMA wants medical treatment for misophonia. Pills baby! Money pal! "Let's drug it up and make a dime off this!"

In navigating the scientific landscape of misophonia, researchers and clinicians strive not only to decode the mysteries of this condition but also to offer tangible support and relief to those whose lives are profoundly influenced by the discordant notes of trigger sounds. As the exploration continues, the hope remains that a more profound understanding will pave the way for effective interventions and, eventually, a comprehensive cure for misophonia. OR... Maybe if everyone would stop chewing loudly and hitting hard "S's," maybe stop being a noisy human. Misophonia wouldn't exist. Too much to ask? Yeah, I thought so.

CHAPTER 5
HOW DO I TELL PEOPLE WHAT I'M DEALING WITH?

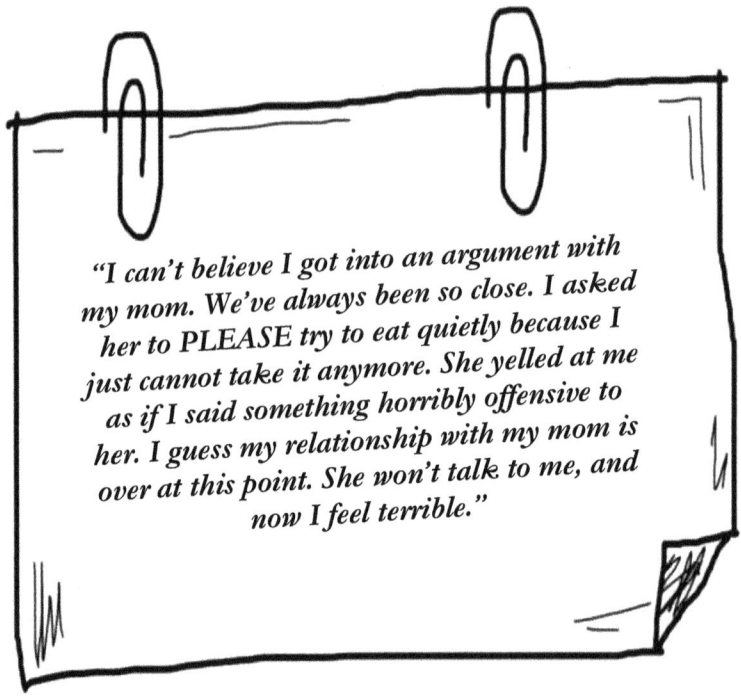

"I can't believe I got into an argument with my mom. We've always been so close. I asked her to PLEASE try to eat quietly because I just cannot take it anymore. She yelled at me as if I said something horribly offensive to her. I guess my relationship with my mom is over at this point. She won't talk to me, and now I feel terrible."

I think I figured it out. I use humor for the most part. Now, I still blurt out stupid things when I'm in the fight or flight stage of dealing with an annoying sound. Yet, I do my very best to either get out of there quickly or crack a joke. "Man, you must be hungry! I can hear you eating from the other room…" or "You're whistling a lovely tune through your nose today; I didn't know boogers were musical instruments." In the best case, they'll realize they're doing it and respectfully quit or attempt to quit making the annoying noise. Like I said to start this off, most of these annoying noise makers have NO IDEA they're even doing it. It's not their fault in most instances.

Now, if you mention it jokingly or poignantly, and they continue to eat like a famished barbarian, then. Well.. they're an asshole. It's as simple as that, folks! "Hey, can you PLEASE not chew so loudly..." "I'll eat any damn way I wanna eat. You don't like it, go away...!" Yeah...at that point, you no longer need to be friends or even related to that person. They don't care about you at all, so leave them in the dust.

Metaphorically, misophonia, like an unruly orchestra, can introduce dissonant notes into the daily symphony of life. Yet, amidst the challenges, individuals with misophonia discover harmonies of coping that allow them to navigate the auditory landscape with resilience and composure.

So here are 20 coping strategies that might or might now work for when you're dealing with someone who doesn't care or understand. Some of these I've used on a daily basis for years.

1. Sound Masking:

Engaging in white noise or calming sounds through headphones or environmental devices can provide a soothing backdrop that helps mask trigger sounds. Ceiling fans, air conditioners, oscillating fans, music, headphones, TV... All saviors!

2. Cognitive Behavioral Therapy (CBT):

CBT techniques, guided by mental health professionals, enable individuals to reframe negative thought patterns and emotional responses associated with trigger sounds. I just recently started reading out for therapy. It's a money-grab system, so I haven't settled on anyone just yet. But I can see how it might help to have someone to speak with. Unless... they hit those hard "Ssssssss." Gah!

3. Mindfulness Meditation:

Embracing mindfulness practices helps individuals stay present in the moment, fostering a non-reactive awareness that can mitigate the impact of trigger sounds. In my humble opinion and abilities, I can't do this. I can't sit still long enough. Due to the tinnitus in my ears from military service, I can't stand it when it's too quiet. But it may work for you.

4. Custom Earplugs:
Specially designed earplugs can offer a personalized solution, allowing individuals to control the volume of incoming sounds without complete isolation.

I have on several instances balled up paper towels or toilet paper and placed it into my ears. It helped, but the ringing in my ears became much louder and equally as terrible as whatever I was hiding from in the first place.

5. Desensitization Exercises:
Gradual exposure to trigger sounds in a controlled and supportive environment, guided by professionals, can help reduce the emotional response over time.

I think this means that we should attempt to get used to it. Can't and won't happen. Not me at least. Nope.

I'm not going to subject myself to some loud lip smacking for hours at a time in an attempt to grow familiar with it. I think I'd rather jump out of a moving car.

6. Support Groups:
Joining support groups or online communities provides a platform for sharing experiences, coping strategies, and emotional support with others facing similar challenges.

Are there misophonia support groups? Maybe online? Hello? Anyone?

7. Healthy Lifestyle Choices:
Maintaining a balanced lifestyle through regular exercise, a nutritious diet, and sufficient sleep can contribute to overall well-being and resilience.

This is a basic cure all for everyone and everything. I'm about 30lbs overweight and I imagine if I lost it I'd feel much better about every aspect of life. But that's a different book.

8. Distraction Techniques:
Engaging in activities that capture attention, such as reading, hobbies, or creative endeavors, can redirect focus away from trigger sounds.

I do this often. I change the tone of the room and change my own volumes and activities. I try to get whoever is making that sound to quit making that sound. If they have a loud phone in their hand, I'll ask them a question, " Hey, can you pause that for a moment..." then ask something I come with on the spot. There's so much that we deal with on an hourly basis. If you know, you know. If you don't, I hope you'll understand.

9. Communication Strategies:

Open and honest communication with friends, family, and colleagues about misophonia helps create understanding and support in various social settings.

This is king. This has helped me so much. Just be honest. "Hey, I really have a mental issue, and I need you to understand this."

Some of my best friends eat like mongoloids, and I can't deal with it. I was stuck in a vehicle with one of my favorite people on Earth recently, and we were headed to film a segment for a movie in Tennessee together. All was good until he pulled out a Tootsie Pop. Now he has blood sugar issues, and I get that. Yes, do what you need to do, man! But a Tootsie Pop in his hands is hours of mind blistering slurping and smacking just 2 feet from my ear.

I wanted to run. I love the guy, so I didn't say anything, but maybe I should have. It just sucked so bad. I never left without headphones on our trips after that.

10. Noise-Canceling Headphones:

High-quality noise-canceling headphones provide an effective barrier against trigger sounds, allowing individuals to create a controlled auditory environment.

It's to quiet for me. But on places, or if music is piping through the headphones, yes.. Much better!

11. Creating Safe Spaces:

Designating specific areas where trigger sounds are minimized or avoided provides a refuge for relaxation and respite.

This is key as well. Right now, I've set up in my mom's office upstairs and away from everyone. I need privacy and a place void of ANY noise made by ANYONE else, no matter how much I love them and love being with them.

12. Employing Technology:
Utilizing smartphone apps or devices that offer customizable ambient sounds or guided relaxation sessions can contribute to emotional regulation.

Often at night, whether I'm in the van or in a house, I play thunderstorm sounds. They relax me and offer up enough white noise in the background to drown out just about everything.

You can find these on apps, Apple Music, or even on YouTube.

13. Establishing Routines:
Predictable routines and structures in daily life create a sense of stability, reducing anxiety related to unexpected trigger sounds.

Doing research on this as a 6 %er in the misophonia realm is eye-opening. Some things are spot on pertaining to my personal struggle, and others have no bearing whatsoever. I'm a non-routined human outside of bruising teeth and taking vitamins, etc. But maybe having better routines can hinder your misophonia issues... maybe? I dunno...

14. Educating Others:
Sharing information about misophonia with friends, family, and colleagues fosters empathy and understanding, leading to more supportive interactions.

Yeah, just wrote a book about it. I'm doing my part. Do yours!

15. Professional Guidance:
Seeking guidance from mental health professionals, audiologists, or specialists in misophonia can provide tailored strategies and coping mechanisms.

As I had previously mentioned, I've been trying. But once I got a taste of how profit crazy these clinics and offices were, it was just a sour taste.

16. Physical Exercise:
Regular physical activity contributes to overall well-being and can be a powerful outlet for releasing built-up tension.

I need to partake more in this option. If I could only figure out how to get into that exercise zone and use it as a release, I think I'd be better off.

17. Art and Expression:
Engaging in artistic pursuits, such as painting, writing, or music, offers a creative channel for emotional expression and catharsis.

Misophonia has been said to be the mark of a creative genius. I write books, film TV shows, act, and film movies, and have a shirt company and a whole streaming TV network called ASY TV. I make coloring books and create a travel app and more. And it does distract me from the daily sounds that bug me. I think there's a lot to this. And I love being called a creative genius.

18. Acceptance and Mindset:
Embracing an acceptance-focused mindset and acknowledging misophonia as part of one's experience can reduce the emotional impact of trigger sounds.

Embracing things... Pain, Loss, Grief, Stress... It's not a choice. You HAVE to embrace these things because you have no option but to embrace them. This one sounds like a psychologist's mumble-jumble. Of course, you're embracing it. But don't be one of those people who use it as their identity. That's so lame. Even if you write a book about it or give speeches to adoring followers, just don't make it your everything. That's what people do when they need attention.

19. Therapeutic Interventions:
Participating in therapeutic interventions like biofeedback or neurofeedback can help individuals gain control over physiological responses to trigger sounds.

It sounds nice and technical. I have no idea what this means. Do you?

20. Pre-Planning for Events:
Before attending events or social gatherings, pre-planning coping strategies, such as having an exit plan or utilizing coping tools, can enhance preparedness.

I do attempt to do this. "Oh, I have a date tonight... I hope she eats quietly." If she doesn't, it'll be a short date. Haha.

These coping strategies form a diverse toolkit, empowering individuals with misophonia to reclaim control over their auditory experiences and foster a sense of well-being in their daily lives.

In intimate personal relationships, the discordant notes of misophonia can introduce challenges that often remain unspoken. Initiating conversations about this intricate condition requires a delicate balance of vulnerability, education, and empathy. So, let's explore how one might navigate these discussions with parents, partners, children, and the rest of the Universe.

Parents:
For many, the journey begins with revealing misophonia to parents. Start by framing the conversation in your personal experiences. Share specific instances where certain sounds trigger intense emotional responses. Use relatable analogies, helping them understand that it's more than a mere irritation; it's an overwhelming emotional reaction rooted in the brain's response to specific sounds.

The Significant Other:
Explaining misophonia to a spouse involves creating a safe space for open communication. Choose a calm moment to discuss your experiences, emphasizing that it's not a critique of their habits but a unique challenge you face. Please encourage them to ask questions and express their feelings while collaboratively exploring coping strategies that work for both of you.

Kids
Discussing misophonia with children requires a gentle approach. Frame the conversation in simple terms, using age-appropriate language. Please encourage them to be mindful of certain behaviors, like chewing with their mouth open, without instilling fear or blame. Emphasize the importance of shared understanding and collaboration as a family.

What Most People Often Misunderstand:
Misophonia's complexity often leads to widespread misunderstanding. People may perceive it as a trivial annoyance rather than a significant challenge. Highlight that misophonia involves an involuntary emotional response, not a choice.

It's not about being overly sensitive but experiencing a heightened reaction to specific sounds that affect daily life and well-being.

A Wider Ignorance:
The need for more awareness of misophonia globally stems from its relatively recent recognition and the intricate nature of its manifestation. Explain that it's an emerging field of study and that conversations like the one you're having contribute to a broader understanding. Encourage curiosity and a willingness to learn about sensory sensitivities.

CHAPTER 6
CAN WE ALL JUST GET ALONG?

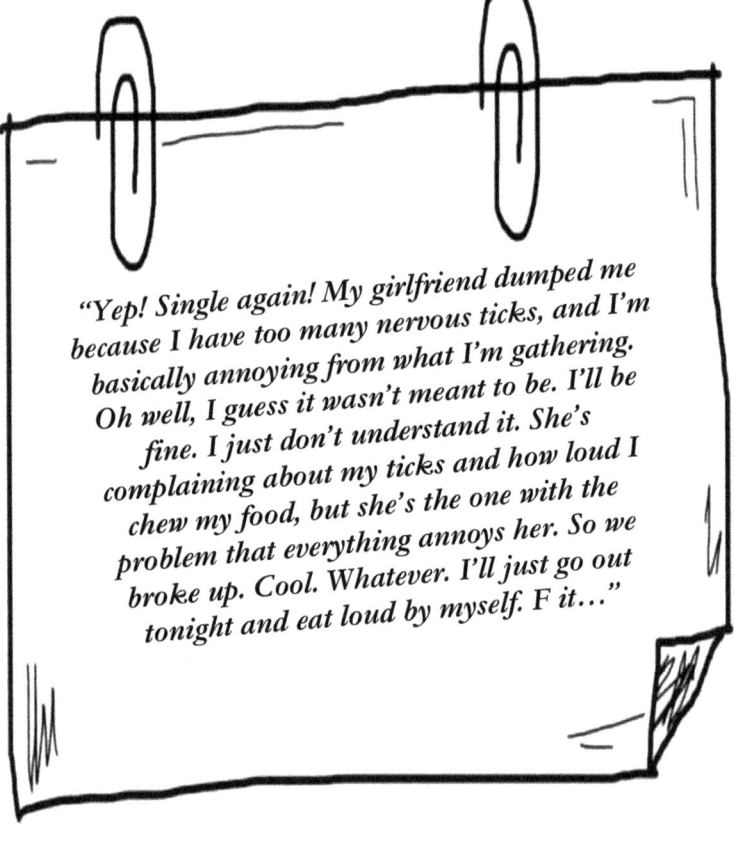

"Yep! Single again! My girlfriend dumped me because I have too many nervous ticks, and I'm basically annoying from what I'm gathering. Oh well, I guess it wasn't meant to be. I'll be fine. I just don't understand it. She's complaining about my ticks and how loud I chew my food, but she's the one with the problem that everything annoys her. So we broke up. Cool. Whatever. I'll just go out tonight and eat loud by myself. F it..."

Can we all just get along? I mean, yeah… I think. Personally, I will never be able to eat with you if you chew loudly. I can't do it, and I won't do it. I don't care if I'm at a once-in-a-lifetime family dinner with all of my best friends and idols around a large, wonderful table filled with all of my lifetime favorite foods. If Mel Brooks and Roger Waters are eating loudly, I'll gobble down as much as I can as fast as I can gobble it and quickly exit the premises. And I hate that...

I want to sit here with everyone I love and idolize. I want to dig deep into their minds and sit under every branch of that learning tree. I want to show my friends and family that I adore spending time with them and create memories that will last longer than I will. But I can't.

In a perfect world, everyone would chew quietly, drive quietly, not endlessly crinkle plastic wrappers, lisp out "S's," and noise pollute neighborhoods with fireworks and leaf blowers.

In a more perfect world, none of this would phase me in the least.

But it's not a perfect world. I'm annoyed to the point of pain and anguish by so many things that straightforward enjoyment is often a problematic realm to reach.

So we move forward and take each case as it comes. "Ah, dogs are going crazy next door. Hmm, the ceiling fan is ticking for some reason; oh, perfect, a little girl across the street is bouncing a basketball on the sidewalk; hey, I hear bass-driven garbage music coming from someone's car out front. Hey, look, the neighbors down the street are getting a new roof. Oh damn, there's a leaf blower, man! No leaves out there, but he's on it! Oh great, now the dog is licking his balls!

FUCK!!!!! ALL I WANTED TO DO I RELAX AND SIP SOME COFFEE ON MY COUCH FOR AN HOUR!!! THAT'S ALL!!!! WHY CAN'T YOU ALL JUST BE FUCKING QUIET FOR ONCE!!!!!!???

And that... is misophonia.

ACKNOWLEDGEMENTS

Thank you so much to Gary Vincent for getting this out there.

Thank you to those who understand what someone with misophonia deals with and attempt to make it easier.

To those who don't care and just carry on with what you're doing, well, you're not the best version of yourself. Don't play a victim, and try being respectful.

To those dealing with Misophonia, be as tolerant as you can be. Choose flight over fight. Inform those you love and people you have constant contact with. And understand it when others don't. Also, be respectful and do your very best to not lose control. I know it's rough.

Thanks to my wonderful mom, Jeanette, and her awesome husband, Ronald. It's been wonderful spending this time with each of you.

RIP, Marci J Cat

Big love to my daughter Charlotte and grandson Chance. So glad you both came into my life.

Miss you, Bear. Can't wait til you come around someday.

Watch ASY TV on roku or at ASYTV.com
Get The AdventureBot Travel App
Check out The HUMAN Shirt Company on Etsy
Find my other books on Amazon.
Watch The ASY TV VANLIFE on Youtube.

www.ingramcontent.com/pod-product-compliance
Lightning Source LLC
Chambersburg PA
CBHW061311040426
42444CB00010B/2598